SPIRIT IS THE JOURNEY

Inspired by Johnny Clegg and Jaluka. The meaning of the lyrics resonate with the authors in a way that symbolizes our own journeys as well as the journeys of the African people of many nations for which the song was originally written.

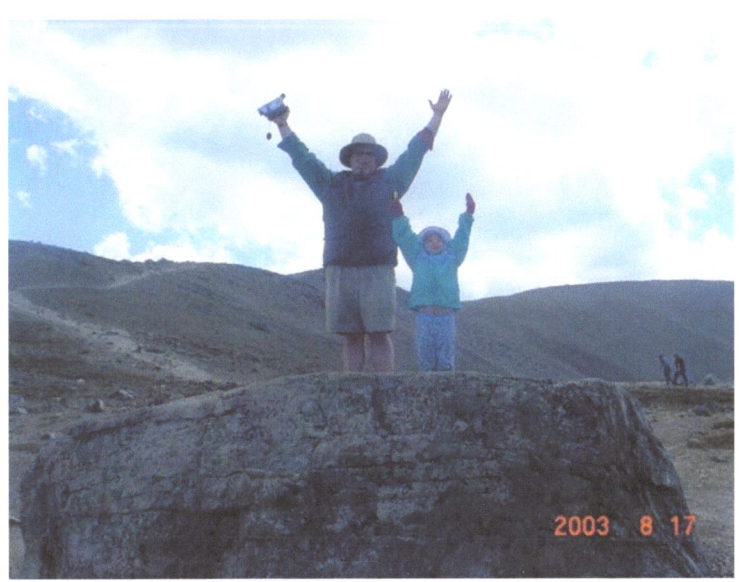

Meara and I at Dinosaur Park, Drumheller Alberta

Spirit Is the Journey
Copyright © 2023 by Mark & Charlotte Maloney

Front Cover Art by:
Kiera Maloney

All rights reserved. No part of this publication may be reproduced, distributed, or transmitted in any form or by any means, including photocopying, recording, or other electronic or mechanical methods, without the prior written permission of the author, except in the case of brief quotations embodied in critical reviews and certain other non-commercial uses permitted by copyright law.

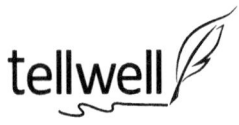

Tellwell Talent
www.tellwell.ca

ISBN
978-0-2288-7377-8 (Paperback)

Dedication

The following writings of my journey would not have been possible without the love and commitment of many people but 2 in particular. These people are, in no particular order, my sister Carolyn Maloney who was my stem-cell donor as well as a huge support throughout my journey. Also, my spouse, Charlotte Maloney, who was with me everyday since my journey began. The things she did for me is a list too big to write here but when things looked really bad she was there to pick me up in any way she could.

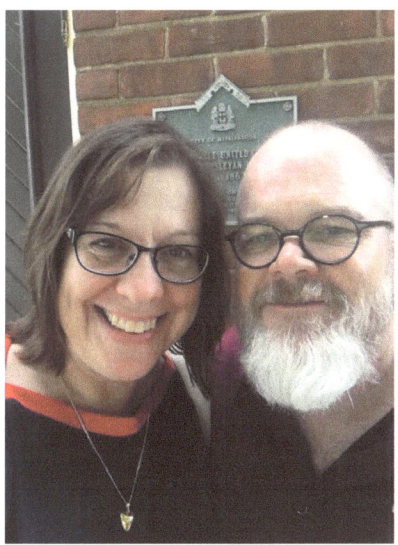

Charlotte and I at the site of our marriage in Mississauga Ont. on our 26th wedding anniversary August 7, 2019

Charlotte

For Sarah, George and Abigayle who never got to tell their own stories but had a profound effect on my life.

Acknowledgements

Mark

There are too many people that are part of my journey to mention by name. I am in awe of the number of people who played a part in my diagnosis, treatment and continuing recovery. Almost all of my time spent in hospital was against the backdrop of the Covid-19 pandemic so I applaud all hospital staff for their service under these circumstances.

First, there is the medical staff at Grand River Hospital, including the Oncology floor (for inpatients) and the attached Cancer Centre (for outpatients). These 2 facilities are staffed with doctors, registered nurse practitioners and nurses but also includes a team that play a very specific role such as pharmacists, social workers, psychologists, imaging, porters, cleaners, food service and others.

I was also a patient at the Hamilton Health Sciences where I spent time at the Hamilton General Hospital (for my back), Juravinski Cancer Centre, and the Juravinski Hospital. The latter is where I spent most of my 183 days as an inpatient. I came across a remarkable staff with extremely high levels of compassion and expertise. Again, there was a team of people who looked after my care including doctors and registered nurse practitioners. They seemed to consider and act upon my condition quickly. There were many nurses, staff from the various teams such as thrombosis, respirology, cardiology, imaging, psychiatry and more.

I also received countless messages from family, extended family, friends, and former colleagues.

To every single one of you I am eternally grateful.

Charlotte

Our daughter Meara was a HUGE support for me through this entire process. It was a scary, uncertain time for all of us in February 2020 and Meara was my source of routine, support, and encouragement. She and I figured out together many of the physical aspects of suddenly being without Mark's strength and knowledge of a ton of tasks for maintaining our house. We figured out how to cut the grass, move furniture, do simple repairs and somehow laughed during it and then felt proud of ourselves when we finished. Meara introduced me to chicken shawarma - an addiction I may have to seek help for at a later time - and we bonded over many late night styrofoam containers of the stuff during Mark's hospitalization.

Meara was forced to grow up so quickly through all of this, and I wish she did not have to say her father having ALL and a stem cell transplant was part of her growing up experience. I am extremely proud of her, and love her dearly.

SPIRIT IS THE JOURNEY

Preface

Mark

This account has multiple purposes, some factual and some emotional. I also sincerely hope it will help other stem-cell transplant patients and their support groups. It gives me a chance to reflect on the journey and learn more about what was happening for the first 22 months after diagnosis. There were long stretches of time when I was not coherent. As a result I don't remember many very difficult periods. Charlotte and Meara have filled in many of those blanks for me and allowed me to realize what a tough road it was for them, my family and all of the staff who looked after me. For patients, the importance of having a primary support person and other family members on top of all of the staff is critically important for a positive outcome.

Second, there are a few defining moments in a person's life; marriage, parenthood and getting or not getting that dream job. For me back in 1997 we were expecting our first child. By all accounts everything was going well until the day she was born. She was critically ill and we had no idea until Sarah was born. She lived for 57 days with Adams-Oliver Syndrome before she passed away. It knocked us off our feet. As we worked through this we realized being her parents would define us in many ways. As a teacher it was a positive thing. I looked at children in my care differently.

I appreciated each one more. Their own children are the most important aspect of the lives of parents and it was up to me to take good care of them. As the years have passed I still think of her as a fighter. The doctors were in awe of how long she survived given the extent of her condition. I was so proud of her. She inspired me to fight Leukemia.

My journey with Leukemia is another defining time.

Charlotte

For myself, the creation of this book began as an opportunity to get Mark "up to speed" with the details and events of the first 22 months. It was an opportunity for us to sit together in the same room during the cold weather at the start of 2021 and piece together events and timelines which Mark was not cognizant of due to his medications and mental state at the time, and the blurring of time which naturally happens with 185+ days as an inpatient in hospital.

I want anyone reading this to know that every event, setback or complication we may talk about was worth it, in my opinion, because as I type this on a sunny, warm spring morning Mark is sitting in the chair beside me in our family room (and he's in good spirits and getting stronger) and that was not something I was guaranteed might happen even 6 months ago.

Every stem cell recipient reacts differently to the process and medications and everyone's unique genetic make-up makes it impossible for medical staff to predict what, if any, complications and reactions an individual might have. Some of the patients who Mark met during induction treatment (a chemotherapy regimen designed to cause remission and a necessary first step on the journey to transplant) at Grand River Hospital he also met with again at Juravinski Oncology Day Services. Each of them had their own experiences - not one of them had the same combination of issues and those who shared a complication, such as mucositis, had it to varying degrees of severity but no two were the same.

Time also softens the many emotions I experienced during critical times. I can think back to Mark's first stint in ICU in August 2020 with less anxiety and a calmer, clearer perspective. It was a huge journey he has been on, and it was a privilege to be by his side and witness his amazing will to live and the fight and determination he displayed. This is HIS experience with stem cell transplant and ALL and our journey together but anyone else walking this path will find their feet don't quite fit into our prints, and they will make their own distinct footprints on this path. The journey is worth it!

THE PLAN

June 2019	Mark retires
June 2019 - June 2023	Mark completes various odd jobs and we complete some updates on the house in preparation for selling it
June 2022	Charlotte retires
June 2026	sell the house, move to a high rise condo
May 2027	buy our second home in PEI
July 2027	spend half the year in PEI and half in Waterloo and live happily ever after

THEN......

Spirit is the Journey

Mark

I was lying in Emergency at 11 p.m. on February 2, 2020. I thought "How bad can this be?". Probably just the usual winter ailments. Then I was visited by an emergency room doctor who told me I had Leukemia. My blood work had revealed malignant white blood cells, or "blasts" as they were also known. I didn't know what a blast was at the time but I knew that Leukemia was cancer of the blood. I felt a sudden wave of what I would later recognize as shock. It seemed to soften the whole moment, as if my cares lessened. It was the strangest sensation I had ever felt. He then went on to tell me "it is 2020 and there are things they can do. You have to stay strong". Those words seemed to resonate with me. I remember them very clearly. I didn't know much about cancer, especially treatments for specific types of cancer. Shortly after that I was being told I was on my way to oncology. A few moments later I saw Charlotte, who had returned with my overnight bag. That was when I told her my diagnosis. I didn't "sugar coat" it, I recall just blurting it out. She always remains stoic at first when being told bad news. This was really bad news. This would be the beginning of a very long and arduous journey for her, Meara, me and the rest of my family. Charlotte has helped in innumerable ways from then to now. So off I went on a bed, down the hall to my hospital room where I would remain for 38 days. I was in a daze, not knowing exactly when treatment would start or how sick I actually was. This is when Charlotte sprung into action and began listening to the doctors and began taking notes. She had a binder that left no stone unturned since I was effectively incoherent from the whole situation in general and the drugs they were beginning to pump into me specifically.

Charlotte was always there but I do also remember a few early visitors such as my brother Kevin, my mom Dianne, my sister Carolyn, my friend John and of course Meara. I remember her the most. I was trying to help her make sense of the fact that I was going to be alright although I really had no clear sense of that at the time. Also, special thanks to my cousin Tracey who was in regular contact with me. She made a trip from Ottawa to Kitchener in my early days of treatment when visitors were still allowed. She brought me a poster that represented thoughts of love and support and photographs of my extended family in the Ottawa area.

Charlotte

Tomorrow is February 2, 2021. A year since Mark's diagnosis. On February 1, 2020 we were on a date in Stratford, shopping for a casserole dish, having dinner at Planet Diner and driving home in a snowstorm oblivious to what was ahead of us. February 2 marked the beginning of a year of profound sadness, profound loneliness and profound helplessness; a year where I cried every day. Some days it was gentle tears going down my face, some days it was "ugly" crying where my eyes and face were red and my nose streamed down my face as much as my tears did, and some days there were tears of joy- on the rare occasion all three occurred on the same day.

But on February 2 it was ugly crying. Leukemia. I was in shock, devastated, speechless, heartbroken and scared. It was 2 a.m. on February 3 when I finally got home and spent the rest of the night lying in the double bed in Gemini's room (Gemini is our rescue dog) sobbing and wailing constantly, so much so that Meara could hear me four floors below in her basement bedroom. She knew it was serious.

Many years ago as a young teenager, my best friend Gail and I had a discussion where I vowed I would never get married unless I met the absolutely perfect person for me- life was too short to be spent with someone who wasn't your soulmate. I think my parents thought they'd be stuck with me until I was in my forties- apparently I could be difficult. Who knew?

When I met Mark I thought I was the luckiest person alive! Finally someone who had similar interests, was very intelligent, could challenge me, had an amazing sense of humour and was incredibly handsome to boot! Finally someone who GOT me, and surprisingly was very accepting of me and actually seemed to like me! Mark is my soulmate. On our wedding day, my maid of honour and best friend Gail was at our house, and we were dressing for the wedding and she looked at me and said -with great frustration- "oh my god, how can you not be nervous?! I'm a nervous wreck!!"

I remember just smiling at her and telling her marrying Mark was the best decision I had ever made and I was completely sure of that.

Now it was February 3, and I was scared shitless. My life partner, my best friend, my soulmate was dying. Me, the eternal control freak, was helpless to do anything to save him. I am not a doctor, I have no medical training and I HATED being so helpless- feeling so weak and scared, so powerless and hopeless. And our daughter!!!! Our beautiful daughter Meara! How could I ever explain to her what was going on with her dad?! I played various speeches and scenarios over in my head, but how do you tell your child their dad is very, seriously ill?

Mark

Rewinding about 7 months, it was July 2019. I felt like I was in a pretty good place in the world. I had a successful marriage, I had just retired after 29 years of teaching and I had a 20 year old daughter of whom we were very proud. The first 5 months after retiring I lived like I had the world by the tail. I thought I could live like this for a long time and decide what my next steps were going to be. I liked the idea of occasional teaching and did that for 4 months.

During that time I started to feel unwell but didn't think too much of it. Upon looking back I realized I had been writing down symptoms that made me feel unwell, from late October until my admission to hospital. I should have paid more attention to them. I was self-diagnosing much lesser ailments. I was experiencing such things as night sweats, insomnia, thirst, low energy and motivation, dizziness and some headaches. Other symptoms included a cough that started in late afternoon, paleness and lack of appetite. Charlotte and Meara were more worried about me than I realized. I was later told that I had mood changes and was not very pleasant at times. I didn't notice this. I did some teaching in January 2020 but things weren't improving. I had purple/red sores appearing in my mouth so I believe that was the turning point for me. Eventually on February 2 I agreed to visit the Emergency department at Grand River Hospital. I thought maybe I had a lung infection or something that could be resolved with antibiotics.

The First Sign

Charlotte

The very first inkling I had that ANYTHING was wrong with Mark was the fall of 2019. It was nothing most people would notice. I have a very acute sense of smell and it was Mark's "smell" which first attracted me to him. And it was Mark's smell which was fading in the fall of 2019 and by December of 2019 was completely absent. This was an indication of something changing with his body chemistry.

Then, in mid December during a conversation before I had to leave for school one weekday morning, I became aware something was wrong. We were hosting the Maloney side for a Christmas gathering and I wanted to phone the butcher shop to order our turkey, so I asked Mark if he had heard how many of his family were coming. The look on his face, and especially in his eyes, was NOT Mark. Nor was his response, which was "What's the matter?! You don't know how to count?!". I was stunned! Mark never spoke to me with such derision. I explained further by asking him if he had had any texts from his family indicating if any members were bringing significant others so I had a final head count. And again, he had that look in his eye (which I would see many times when he was hallucinating in the ICU) and he said "Are you stupid?! Can't you count?!".

Now I had tears going down my face and told him, as calmly as I could muster, "Do not speak to me like that." but by now, the look was gone from his face and his eyes were clear. Now he looked stunned and asked why I was crying. I repeated his words to him and he looked appalled and completely denied ever saying that. I was worried it was early onset dementia- little did I know.

Mark

As I look back, gratitude prevails. I was diagnosed right in the emergency room. Treatment started soon afterwards. I was diagnosed specifically with Acute Lymphoblastic Leukaemia, B-Cell (ALL). This is a type of Leukaemia that is most often found in paediatrics. My case was fairly unusual and I had an unusual and complex chromosomal abnormality. There are many causes that are possible for Leukemia. I was told that mine was most likely a mutation. I have no history of this illness in my family to which I am aware.

The treatment was fast and aggressive. I was really incoherent at the time but Charlotte was always there to take notes and fully understand the gravity of the situation. I was able to continue to have visitors then as it was before the pandemic, or Covid-19, began to close in on the world.

Charlotte

I cannot remember the specific date, but I do know it was a weekday - early in the week so Monday or Tuesday - and it was February 2020, midmorning. It was a cold but sunny winter day, Mark was sleeping in his hospital bed as the bag of platelets dripped into his veins. He had received units of blood, platelets and plasma for several days in a row, depending on the results of his daily 5 a.m. bloodwork. I was in awe, and extremely grateful that no matter which product was needed - blood, platelets or plasma - they were produced and infused within a few hours of his CBC being done. I texted a friend of mine to share my thoughts on how fortunate we were to be in Ontario and have access to safe and seemingly abundant blood products, and how it would be so great to be able to "pay it forward". She happened to be on her planning time (my friend is also a colleague) and she responded right away in agreement. Then she texted me again about 20 minutes later to tell me she was going to host a blood drive in Mark's name at our local Canadian Blood Services Clinic. She had contacted several "recruiters" who were friends of ours at various schools in our local board. They had 50 slots for people to sign up to be tested/donate. Our daughter also contacted some of her friends, especially those who knew her dad and some had even been his students. The original idea had been to decorate the clinic, bring food and drink, and Meara and I would be there in person to thank donors - a bit of a party atmosphere to celebrate the contribution everyone was making. Covid 19 shut down that idea, but everyone who signed up was able to go donate and we had to make due with a letter Mark wrote (see Appendix A) to all those donating in his honour being posted at the sign-in desk. I know several of those who donated that day have continued to do so every three months. We are eternally grateful and thankful for their donating and for our friend Jan who organized the blood drive.

Mark

The fine staff at Grand River Hospital in Kitchener were able to get me into remission. That was the first step on this journey. I was released from hospital 38 days later. I would continue with chemotherapy on an out-patient basis until the end of June 2020. This required 2 or 3 visits weekly to the hospital plus taking chemotherapy medication at home. The visits as an out-patient usually took most of a day. By the time I had blood work done, and the drugs were prepared, administered, and the associated waiting, 4-6 hours would pass. The staff there were kind but those were difficult days.

The months at home were challenging. Chemotherapy uses very powerful drugs that made me very unwell most of the time. As I had always heard, chemotherapy was in itself very difficult and hard on the body. I had what became known in our household as "Chemo Brain". I also felt significant anxiety and loss of appetite. I wasn't myself which was very hard on Charlotte and Meara as well as me. I was also very weak. Walking became very difficult. I became weaker over the period of time I was on chemotherapy.

One thing I was not expecting were weak bones. It turns out my back was very weak from Osteoporosis and Spinal Stenosis. Apparently I had been living with both conditions for a long time. I was told this by my Orthopedic surgeon after an emergency MRI at Juravinski Hospital. The L4 vertebrae probably collapsed at least 2 years before. The surgeon who looked at my x-rays said he didn't know how I wasn't a parapelegic. Towards the end of June I had x-rays that showed a new fracture in L1. No wonder I was in so much pain. Later in the summer an additional fracture was revealed, T5. It was determined that I was eligible to have the stem-cell transplant. I was told sometime in April that I was a candidate for this procedure so I just kept looking forward, not to let back pain get in the way of this life-saving treatment. Once approved for the transplant, I had to wait until I was deemed ready to have the procedure. I wasn't nearly ready in mid-April. I would continue with chemotherapy until late June. There was no other long term alternative to which I was aware. The goal was a cure so I carried on with the treatment.

STEM-CELL TRANSPLANT

I was told early on at Grand River Hospital that once I was in remission an Allogeneic Stem-Cell Transplant was my best chance at longer term survival. Allogeneic meaning I needed a stem-cell donor. Stem-cells are located in bone marrow. They can become whatever is needed. In my case they needed to become red and white blood cells as well as platelets. I was fortunate to have 3 siblings who were most likely to provide a close match. I have 2 brothers and a sister all in their fifties like me. All 3 were quite willing to get tested. I was grateful at their willingness to become involved in this life saving process. As it turns out it was more likely that my sister would provide the closest match since females usually provide the best match. My sister agreed to be my donor. Special thanks to the 3 of them. My sister literally saved my life.

Finding a Stem Cell Donor - It started on February 5, 2020

Charlotte

I was not familiar with any of the specifics regarding stem cell transplants when Mark's oncologist asked to speak to me in the hall at Grand River Hospital on the morning of February 5, 2020. She asked me to verify the information Mark had given her the day before - he had three siblings, their ages and sexes. She wanted further detail from me - where they lived, what they did for a living, family situation, their exercise and lifestyle habits. The fact he had a sister was a positive - females and our double X make us very compatible donors if all other factors matched.

I was given the Coles' notes version of being a potential stem cell donor. Blood samples would be taken and analyzed for Human Leukocyte Antigens, matches would need to be very close (at least an 8/10) and donation would not be much different than donating blood. Should his brother in British Columbia be a match, the Ontario government would look after flying him in for donation. I was then given a sheet of paper and asked to contact his siblings, any living parents and offspring to see if they would agree to be screened and fill in their information on the sheet which would be forwarded to the stem cell program at Juravinski Hospital immediately. That was all.

So off I went to the lounge area on the oncology ward with this simple piece of paper and my pen. I believe I called Kevin first. I remember telling him siblings had the greatest potential to be a donor for a stem cell transplant, it would mean he needed to have a blood test and if he was a match he could decide if he wanted to go through with it or not. Unlike bone marrow donation, stem cell donation was just like giving blood and not a surgical procedure. I remember Kevin didn't even hesitate for a minute, but said to sign him up and would it help if he came to the hospital right now. I told him I only needed contact information and his birthdate, and asked if he wanted to talk to his wife Leanne about this first and think about it. He explained if it was going to save Mark's life then what was there to think about, just sign him up!

Next I called his brother Paul in B.C.. Paul worked various shifts in Fort McMurray but lived in Revelstoke and my call fortunately found him at home with some time to chat. Paul was just as quick as Kevin to give me his information. He was concerned the fact he lived in B.C. might delay determining if he was a match. As it turns out, Mark's oncologist gave me the specific test names needed, and where the blood needed to be sent. Paul walked into his local hospital and told them what he needed done and why, and 48 hours later his blood was in Hamilton.

Last I called his sister Carolyn who was at work but between clients and had a bit of time to take my call. She, like her older brothers, did not hesitate to consent. I also told her being female made the chances of her being a potential match higher - a fact which turned out to be true.

It was April 22, 2020 when the head of his Hematology team shared the news with Mark (and myself via a conference phone call from the parking lot thanks to Covid) that his sister was a very strong match!!!!

I so clearly recall how willingly and selflessly all three of Mark's siblings volunteered to be donors. I am eternally grateful to all three of them for being so brave and willing to save Mark's life. I remember shaking, and feeling overwhelmed and unsure of myself when I entered the lounge knowing I had to make three phone calls to ask them to make such a sacrifice, and how I felt so elated and humbled by their quick and positive responses. Carolyn was ultimately the match, and she endured emotional and physical distress by agreeing to do so, but I am forever thankful to Kevin, Paul and Carolyn for all readily agreeing to possibly be the donor out of their love for their brother.

I would also like to mention that although there was only a 25% chance of being a match, our daughter Meara was adamant she be listed as a potential donor for screening. If none of his siblings were a match, Meara would have been tested as a potential donor. The stem cell transplant team would also have begun looking through the international stem cell donor list for a match. Our daughter Meara has now registered with the international donor list, as she witnessed how her father's life was saved by having a transplant and she would like to be able to offer the same to another individual.

Mark

July 22- Carolyn's donation

My sister Carolyn attended the hospital several times leading to donation day. She underwent several tests and meetings to confirm that she was a viable donor. I was able to visit her on the day she was donating her cells. This procedure took all day. She felt unwell for about the next 2 weeks. I didn't realize at the time that it would be so physically hard on her, emotional stress notwithstanding. How do you thank someone for this? I'm still trying to figure that out. At that point I was just relieved she was ok.

Carolyn

Finding out my oldest brother Mark had cancer was devastating. Finding out I was a match for stem cell donation was exciting.

Watching my brother go through months of treatment with the strength of a soldier it was the very least I could do to help move him forward in his battle.

Receiving the news that you are a match for stem cell donation is a wonderful experience. It means that you get to give someone a second chance at life.

There were a number of tests that I had to go through to confirm that I was a good candidate. All of these tests pale in comparison to what my brother had to endure during the treatment of his cancer. I am so grateful that I was able to help.

Mark had and still has the most wonderful supportive wife anyone could ask for. Charlotte has been by his side through diagnosis, treatment and remains strong on the other side of Mark's transplant with her care, compassion and overall strength and support.

Considering Mark's course of treatment fell during the pandemic I felt limited in what I could offer as far as help and support, as during Covid the hospitals were limiting and eliminating visitors. I found one of the things I could do was make food and deliver it to the hospital for Charlotte. The hospital had a lounge area with a fridge and microwave for caregivers. It was important to me to contribute something as they were going through so much themselves.

My Christmas wish that year was for Mark to be released from hospital and so it was granted.

Today, the battle continues. Mark makes improvements everyday, and Charlotte still stands by his side.

I must also mention what a relief it is to the rest of the family to have such a strong woman as Charlotte see Mark through his treatment.

Mark

July 23 to July 30

My readiness to enter Juravinski Hospital to begin the process was determined to be July 23. There was significant chemotherapy and other drugs to prepare me for the stem-cell transplant. As you may already guess, this made me feel unwell. After a week the day finally arrived for the procedure to take place. I wouldn't call it surgery. I was fully conscious and the new stem-cells were injected intravenously. It was an emotional time. I had actually gotten to this point in my overall journey. As I look back on my text messages that day, I was elated but not making sense.

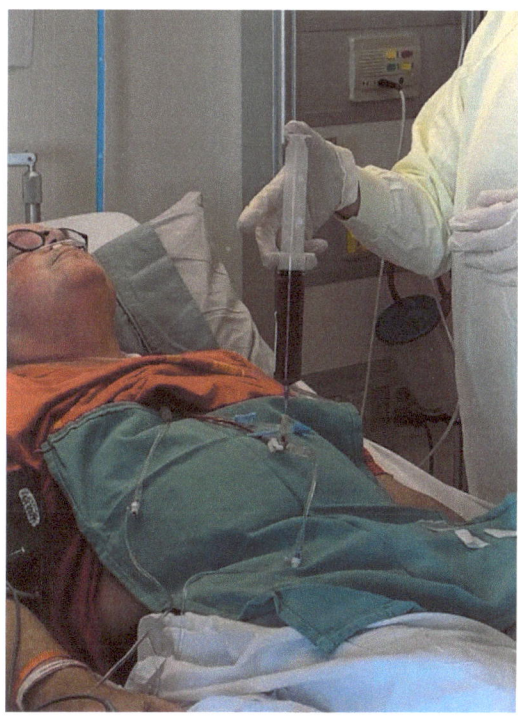

Stem-Cells being injected intravenously. There were five tubes of Carolyn's stem cells- July 30, 2020

Day +1-Day +8

Over the next week things began to get more difficult. Side effects weren't far behind. Mucositis was a major one for me. My own bacteria created an infection. I became very confused, delusional and had many hallucinations. I have memories and stories that occurred during this delusional period. The cocktail of drugs I was taking also contributed to my delusional state. I can recall most of my hallucinations but none of them were real. One example that happened during this time is as follows. I was at the last school at which I taught. It was a Sunday. The building was empty except for 1 English Language Learner (ELL) student and me. She was looking for the ELL teacher and we were somehow in her classroom. The teacher then appeared in her classroom but something was wrong. She leaned against the wall, then slid down the wall to a seated position. I'm told the actual time was about midnight. I panicked, then used my cell phone to call the teacher, Charlotte and 911. The situation was straightened out somehow without Emergency Services (EMS) coming to what I thought was the school, needlessly. It felt so real and I was quite rattled in my delusional world. This was before I was taken to ICU. On August 10 I was taken to the Intensive Care Unit (ICU) where I stayed for 4 days. Once I left ICU I remained confused and was hallucinating for about 6 weeks afterwards. I remember parts of that time period but Charlotte and Meara have clarity in that regard and filled me in on some of the language and behaviour I exhibited during this time. While in ICU, it was shocking to me that I would say and do such nasty things. I swore constantly, was uncooperative and needed to be restrained.

I don't remember any of the staff who helped me during this time. I hardly slept, my mouth was moving with no sounds coming out, my fingers and hands were moving and there were restraints around my waist and wrists. I thought my friend Jim and other people were in the room with me, and I got angry if Charlotte tried to correct me. I remember none of this. Post ICU there are many stories of what I thought was happening at the time such as the one that occurred in what I thought was the school. There were many other examples of stories in my head that were not real. Most of them were not pleasant and some were just frightening. I called 911 a few more times. Most had at least 1 person in them that I knew.

One more example, while I was always in my hospital bed, on dozens of occasions, it seemed like my room was a cube that was turning. I felt like my bed was on a wall or the ceiling and I would fall out if I moved. My room could also be moving around the hospital as one self-contained unit. Another example is the characters in the framed photographs, such as Charlotte, Meara and our dog Gemini, were moving. I also thought I was visiting a secret social club run by a teacher friend and her husband. There were lots of couches and food being served and everyone was having a good time. Sometimes however I was left in a weird holding area. There were eyes periodically peering through the wall as if I was covertly being observed. All of my delusions happened while I was in the hospital. I have heard of patients experiencing delusional behaviour at home which would be that much more difficult. I have, since I got home, been filled in on some of the behaviour and language. Thank-you to everyone who dealt with a highly delusional me.

Charlotte

August was the lowest point I have ever experienced in my life. I have lost loved ones, I have had disappointments, I have lost my daughter Sarah but August was the loneliest I have ever felt in my life. I would like to apologize to our daughter Meara. During this time I was not the mother and support she needed, and for this I will be eternally guilty. I love Meara more than anything but I did not have the capacity to meet Mark's needs in my role as his formal caregiver, and as his wife and still be the mom I wanted to be. I was exhausted and my stress and lack of sleep caused huge issues with my own blood sugar causing me to feel unwell most days. I hope Meara will understand with time that I was trying to help save her dad so she wouldn't be without him. I am just disappointed in myself that this meant she had to temporarily be without her dad AND her mom.

I don't think I would have survived August without the support of my best friend Gail. Covid be damned, she was there for me, wearing a mask. The first night Mark was in ICU she showed up at our house at ten o'clock at night with Tim Hortons and she just listened as we sat there, six feet apart, me sobbing and probably babbling incoherently the whole time.

Mark had begun to "not be himself" shortly after the transplant. Delirium and hallucinations started. At first staff seemed unsure if it was a reaction to the cocktail of drugs he was taking or something else. It turned out to be a blood infection caused by the mucositis, and an interaction between some of his medications. He would "see" things that were not there and he had started to phone me in the middle of the night, as well as some of his colleagues, as the scary situations he was experiencing seemed very real. Medical staff asked me to take his phone and Apple Watch as he also called 911 on several occasions. This was also the time period when his MRI revealed three compression fractures in his back and he was bed ridden- a very disorienting situation as well.

He was moved to ICU on August 10th to treat his severe mucositis as well as provide the necessary supervision for his delirium. A phone call from his nurse at 8 am asking me if I was driving yet made me quickly realize how serious this situation was.

The ICU was a fantastic, well equipped, and new facility. His mental decline was quick and he was restrained in his bed within 24 hours. The staff - and there is a large staff caring for the patients in ICU - were very thorough and extremely knowledgeable. I was Mark's primary caregiver and had power of attorney for care. Suddenly any decisions for his care were mine to make and it was my signature on the stack of papers Mark's doctor brought with him that was needed as Mark no longer had the mental clarity to do so himself. Staff had assessed Mark and deemed him unable to communicate his needs, including whether he was in pain or not, so I was now "calling the shots". Visiting hours were 9 until 8 and the staff wanted me present at 9, as they so delicately explained to me when I arrived at 9:45 a.m. one day, as the doctors needed me there to sign off on procedures (for example, giving him any blood products, removing the infected Hickman, tube feeding him). The nurses said hearing my voice slowed his heart rate down and made him calmer. I had no proof of this though as he often didn't recognize me, and my usually sweet, kind and loving husband berated me up and down and told me to F-off at least a 100 times a day. If I dared to let my emotions show he would call me "soft", a "wuss" and tell me I needed to buck up. I was so afraid he was going to remember all of this, end up hating me, and want a divorce when he got out of the ICU!

I was so scared he was not going to make it. I felt burdened by having to make decisions about his care, look after our finances, try to be a support for our daughter, look after the house and the dog to some degree, deal with the loneliness of not having anyone to reassure me things would be okay, and deal with grieving about having to take early retirement. I felt my retirement was overlooked by some, and the emotional toll it took on me surprised me. I had loved my job and hoped I had made an impact on some of my students, and I was left feeling deflated and insignificant, especially because I did not get to say goodbye to any of them. The death of one of my students in December of 2020 still bothers me greatly. I simply "disappeared" over the Superbowl weekend in February.

Back to Gail, she was my strongest support during this difficult time. My parents were in contact daily, my sister sent food and we talked often, a fantastic neighbour, Sue, became a foster mom to our dog, but Gail was my confidante in what was really troubling me. I had broken two toes in August - I am notoriously clumsy - and they were painful. Gail would check in with me to see how they were healing. Then, when I was in a car accident and on the 401 going to Hamilton one rainy Sunday in August, it was Gail who looked over my handy work at repairing the scratches myself and listened to my story of how I parked in the garage and "hid" it from Meara until I had the time to fix it. Meara feared I might get killed in an accident driving back and forth to Hamilton each day, and then she'd be without a mom and a dad, so I never told. I never called the man's insurance because the car looked fine and I could not mentally handle having to get a rental, get estimates, go through insurance when I just needed to be in Hamilton every day and ensure Mark got better. Nothing mattered except Mark's health. I was very stressed and I felt very alone dealing with "everything". I SO appreciated Gail's frequent check ins, her video calls, and I was dreading September and school starting up as Gail is a teacher and I would miss having her support at my beck and call.

Mark

Day +9- Day + 66

I remained in my current room until about the middle of September. Throughout that time I was confused and belligerent and my back pain got so bad that I became bed-ridden and I lost my mobility. When they eventually thought I could leave the Hematology ward I was transferred to the rehabilitation ward where I would stay for about 3 weeks.

Back pain caused my rehabilitation to be shut down in favour of back surgery.

Day +67-+80

I was taken to Hamilton General Hospital early on the morning of October 5. Surgery was performed to fuse my T12 vertebrae to my L2 using a rod and 4 screws. Despite needing more surgery at the time to repair 2 other vertebrae, I had lost so much blood that the surgeon didn't have the time to continue. I still had at least 2 more fractured vertebrae. Whether I need more back surgery in the future remains an unanswered question at this point. Following surgery I was taken to the hospital's ICU which was standard procedure for the situation. I remained sedated until the next day. I didn't realize I would be sedated that long even though they told me, I didn't internalize it. I was sedated for about 36 hours which was very disorienting. The back surgery completed was successful though. I was to be transferred to the "spine wing" for recovery after a couple of more days when a bed became available. I stayed there for 10 days.

Day +81-Day +98

I was transferred back to the rehabilitation floor at Juravinski Hospital to regain my mobility. I was seen by Physiotherapists and Occupational therapists about 3 times daily. I would make progress to a point where I was released from the hospital to continue my recovery at home. It wasn't long before I could navigate the whole house including the upstairs bedroom. I needed to navigate a 5 step staircase and a 10 step staircase. I didn't bother with the basement and didn't go down those stairs until July 2021.

Day +99-Day +109

While at home I still needed to visit the hospital twice weekly. It was called Oncology Day Services (ODS). I went there 3 times. At my third visit there (November 15) I was diagnosed with another potentially serious side effect called Graft vs Host (GVH) disease. Initially it showed up on the skin but on my third visit to ODS it was determined that the GVH had found its way into my Gastrointestinal Tract. On that visit I complained of nausea, vomiting, lack of appetite, diarrhea and general weakness. I was readmitted to the hospital where I would stay for another 37 days.

Day +109- Day +146

The GVH was very challenging. I was in bed most of the time so I lost whatever mobility I had regained up to that point. This was especially difficult because I had significantly reduced control of my bowels. Charlotte and the hospital staff were very supportive during this very difficult time. I also felt very weak and just wanted to stay in bed. I was told feeling really unwell was part of the process and I would eventually start to feel better. Eventually and slowly I did. Physiotherapy continued through all of this but I was left significantly weaker now than when I was released from Hamilton the first time. I really wanted to get home for Christmas so I was extra motivated. Altogether I had spent about 185 days in the hospital in 2020.

There was another factor at play here and that was a second wave of Covid-19. By all accounts it was worse than the first and it seemed to be affecting many parts of the hospital. The hospital became locked down more tightly as time passed. Charlotte and I got our wish- on December 22 (Day +146) I was released from the hospital again. I was not nearly as strong as I was the previous time I was released but Covid-19 and the holiday shutdown helped in deciding on my release. I would continue to recover at home. I was quite dependent on my caregiver Charlotte for most things at this point but being at home would hopefully help in my recovery and it did. I got more sleep, home cooked meals, the company of my dog Gemini, more privacy and many other things.

December 22- December 31

I was elated to get home. I was so appreciative of the little things. The house was decorated inside and out with lights, other decorations and of course our Christmas tree. Charlotte had gone to great effort late at night to make it special. I enjoyed the gently falling snow, our dog Gemini's welcome and ongoing desire to be close by. It was a happy day for Charlotte too. No more daily drives to Hamilton that took so much of her energy and time. Most importantly, Meara was home Christmas Eve and Christmas Day to visit, open a few presents and share meals. Covid-19 precluded any larger family gatherings. Such was the reality of 2020 and on into 2021 so far.

2021

Mom's contribution

My son has Leukemia! I've just been informed by my #2 son, Kevin that my #1 son, Mark has Leukemia. It was Feb 4, 2020. I was shocked and very worried as our family didn't have serious illnesses like this! Of course I have heard about Leukemia but really knew very little but over the last year have come to know a lot.

Then in March COVID-19 hit and we were all locked down so we couldn't visit much in the hospital. This is when I seriously learned to "FaceTime". So lucky to have this technology to visit and we do often.

Later it was decided Mark would be a good candidate for a Stem Cell transplant so his 3 siblings, Kevin, Paul (my #3 son), and Carolyn were tested for a match. His sister turned out to be a very good candidate and this was planned for the end of July. It wasn't as easy as it sounds and she had to go for considerable testing but it all turned out successful.

However, for Mark there were considerable set backs and he was so sick with Chemo, Mucositis, Graft Versus Host Disease, and back surgery. Carolyn and I sat on the couch and cried wondering if he was going to make it.

Mark had a wonderful, hopeful attitude and a remarkable wife and we believe it was Charlotte as well as the doctors that pulled him through. I had many family and friends praying for his recovery which was also helpful to me.

He came home 2 days before Christmas and is now working on gaining his strength back after a gruelling year of treatment.

Love, Mom 💕 Jan 28, 2021

PS When, this Pandemic is all over, we must have a celebration 🎉 for Mark's recovery and Charlotte's retirement 😇 as unfortunately it got missed in all this confusion.

Mark

I consider my ongoing recovery as being broken roughly into 2 parts; mental/emotional and physical. They don't necessarily recover at the same rate or stay in sync with each other. For me mental clarity was recovering at a faster rate as I understood it at the time. An old saying I remember as a young athlete was "the mind says go but the body says no." This was the case for me. Longer term emotional challenges were starting to become more apparent. More on that later. Physical progress was very slow. After 40 days I spent most of my time on one level of the house where there was a bathroom, television, chairs and a bed had been set up there. I could leave the house through the sliding back door as long as there was a wheel chair outside the door which would get me around to the front of the house, into the car and off to medical appointments. There was little other travel since Covid-19 had its grip on the globe. Charlotte cooked all my meals up to this point and brought them to me in the family room.

Exercise is so important in facilitating my recovery. I was given muscle building exercises and walking as much as possible was also critical. However there were a few main factors that I believe limited my progress during this time. One was my very limited space to walk. It was winter so it wasn't safe to walk outside so I did laps in the family room. I also had a Physiotherapist assigned to me who was showing me how to strengthen my body to increase mobility. More than that however were powerful drugs that were still needed to ward off GVH disease. Specifically Prednisone, a steroid which had great benefits but also many harsh side effects. Slowing down my ability to build muscle and strength as well as weakening the Adrenal gland's ability to produce my own steroids were the biggest side effects for me. By mid-January it was decided that I could begin to reduce the amount of that drug slowly and it would take at least 4 months to wean off this drug. However, by November 2021 I am still taking small amounts. If I went too quickly in discontinuing this drug I risked not being rid of GVH so I had to be patient with this. It has worked so far. I am slowly getting stronger and more independent.

After 4 weeks of being home I could now climb the 5 stairs it takes to get to the next level of the house. It gave me different options as to where I could sit, it allowed me more space to walk and the kitchen is on this level too. I have also been working on independence in the bathroom, getting dressed and standing up from different heights. Each time I improved any of these things, it was considered a milestone of progress.

Along the way since I've been home, I've been hoping my physical progress would get faster, since my brain wanted me to do more. I wanted to walk the dog, cook and eat in the kitchen, shovel the patio, make Charlotte's life easier and many other things that help me transition back to a normal existence.

As I developed more mental clarity I began to become aware of the world around me and was regaining some of my interests and concerns. I hadn't watched television in a year and hadn't spent much time online. I did use text and email a lot to communicate with many people who were providing so much support. I had phone calls too. I am extremely grateful for every one of those messages.

I mostly watched news and sports. Covid-19 and chaos in the United States were the 2 main stories at this time. Covid-19 was keeping me home regardless of whether I was a recovering Leukemia patient or not. So I watched a lot of hockey which I was really enjoying. There wasn't any hockey to watch for a long time. I didn't seem to care for a long time but now I did. It feels really good to look forward to games specifically and plan for the future generally.

Charlotte

The Caregiver Agreement

It was a three page document, it had to be signed by Mark but I can't recall if I had to sign it. It was the caregiver agreement. Mark could not have the transplant without naming a caregiver. I have rarely spoken to anyone outside the medical community about the caregiver agreement. Being his caregiver is at the heart of my trauma diagnosis. I have had conversations with his medical team that you only see played out, like a bad nightmare, on TV. I have had to sign numerous papers consenting to medical procedures, blood products, use of physical restraints, and resuscitation orders. I have been present for numerous spinal taps, bone marrow aspirations and the actual transplant. I have changed numerous bandages, and numerous bed pans, and been an advocate for his care and treatment in numerous medical settings. Thank you Mark for trusting me to make those choices on your behalf! Being his caregiver involved more responsibility for his care and well being, and accountability to his medical team, then I think either of us had realized at the time. Mark is healing and he is here with us - if he didn't have the transplant he would not be here - so I would volunteer to be his caregiver again without hesitation.

Mark

It is now April 5, 2021. I developed a rash over the weekend. I was really concerned that Graft versus Host disease of the skin was returning and could potentially end up back in my Gastrointestinal tract. I made a call to the Hematologist on-call this long weekend. I ended up going to Hamilton that day so the doctor could see my skin. He increased my Prednisone, did bloodwork and passed on the details of my visit to the head doctor of my transplant team and I went home. I dreaded the idea of another readmission to hospital but it thankfully didn't happen. I seemed to feel better as the day went on, especially after increasing my dose of Prednisone. I went back to the hospital a few days later for bloodwork and for my skin to be examined by my medical team. It turns out that the dots on my skin were not a return of GVH. All other indicators, including bloodwork, showed that my recovery was continuing to progress.

The other important thing to remember at this time was that I was feeling better. I felt recent gains in strength and mobility. Charlotte says too that she sees improvements in my mental clarity and that I'm more myself.

Mark

Emotional support in the short term is seen through this writing so far. I was told many times that strong support from my primary caregiver and others was a great indicator for a positive outcome of my journey. I really do believe this to be true. As I think back there are so many examples of Charlotte and others sticking with me when things got excessively difficult for me and her. I also saw many examples of people in the hospitals who had little or no support. I felt very lucky (believe it or not) because I wasn't on my journey alone.

Emotional support also means that councillors are available to talk with Charlotte, I and any others close to me that need to unpack the emotional trauma that has been part of this journey. It is critical to have access to people who can confidentially listen and provide suggestions about how to cope and move forward. For some, it's extremely difficult to revisit these most difficult times. I do believe that it's very helpful to ultimately deal with the trauma. I don't believe trying to just move forward without talking about emotional trauma is helpful. Everyone is different but everyone still suffers.

As the winter went on I began to think about the longer term implications of my journey. I was told that at some point I would fully recover from both the Leukemia treatments and my back pain and mobility issues. I just have to be patient and do as the experts instruct.

It's now May 2 and the journey to recovery continues. It is taking longer than we expected but I have had 3 significant setbacks; Mucositis, GVH of the gastrointestinal tract and a fungal infection in my lungs. It caused a lot of coughing, shortness of breath,"gagging," and general weakness. I developed a fever which is something that needs to be addressed quickly considering we weren't completely sure of its origin. Some thought it may be some form of GVH. Antibiotics solved the fever and a puffer was also prescribed to get the coughing under control. It is taking some time for the puffer to work.

I am also using a drug-free device called "Aerobika." I blow into this device and it provides some resistance to my lungs. The goal is to strengthen and expand my lungs. As it turned out all of my back issues caused me to lose height. I am now 12 centimetres shorter than my peak height when I was young. This caused my left lung to become somewhat compressed at the bottom. Working to expand the volume of my lungs is an on-going goal.

Back to my lung infection which was a separate issue from the lung compression. This was another set back. The symptoms worsened and I was readmitted to hospital again on June 7 to figure out the root of this problem. I stayed for another 5 days to undergo tests. It turned out to be, as I mentioned, a fungus infection in my lungs. The drug I am taking for this infection is a 3-6 month course which is not without its own side effects.

There is also the issue of on-going back pain. This makes everything harder of course. My L4 vertebra (second from the bottom of my spinal cord) remains untreated. I have been trying to strengthen my core muscles to take some stress off my spine. Spinal Stenosis is causing a lack of blood flow to those muscles so there are limits in how strong my core will ultimately be. This damage to my spine predates my Leukemia diagnosis so I already had a weak back.

Walking is a vitally important form of exercise. Re-learning how to walk with a proper gait and posture will strengthen those muscles in my back and take pressure off my spine. I use a walker, walking sticks/poles and a cane. The walking poles I believe give me the best chance to develop a proper gait and posture. I use them outside. It started off very painful and slow but I am improving with them. If I need a break from them, I revert to the walker or cane, especially indoors. I need to use the cane on the stairs at all times at this point. When exercising my back muscles I need to ensure I have "days off" to allow my body to rest and recharge. I don't know at this point if and when I will have more back surgery. Time will tell.

The length of time for recovery becomes very difficult at times. Charlotte and I are finding it very challenging at times. I try to support her in any way I can. I encourage her to talk to others such as friends and counsellors. Currently the government of Ontario has another "stay at home" order in place so there aren't really any options for Charlotte to take such as going anywhere with a friend. It's hard on me to see Charlotte struggle at times but I understand the need to be aware of it. We have an understanding that when 1 of us is having an exceedingly difficult day we let the other know so we can adjust our expectations of each other for the day. Hopefully when Covid restrictions loosen and Ontario gets much better control of the situation, Charlotte will have more options for balance in her life.

As I talked more with Meara I also learned more about the significant emotional challenges she endured, especially while I was incoherent. She is very traumatized by the whole ordeal. I learn a little bit more about how she feels each time she shares. I am very appreciative of her speaking about her trauma. I hope talking and the passage of time will be helpful for her as well. During this time she made me aware of how often she visited with Carolyn. I am so grateful that she had a place to go to get support. This was another example of how family stepped up to help and I didn't become aware of this until recently. I think communication is so important because I didn't understand everything that was going on around me at the time and the toll it takes on people. For me things continue to get better but a lot of trauma and scars still exist for those around me.

Also on May 2, I got my second Covid vaccination. I was put on a priority list due to my status as a stem-cell transplant recipient. I am grateful for that. Only about 2% of Ontario's population has been vaccinated at this point in time. All went well with both doses.

The other significant issue for me is, will the Leukemia return and when? As of the summer I am not really that worried about it and no one really knows the answer to either part of that question. One way to look at it is to realize that no one really knows their life expectancy. I have more significant risk factors but in the end no one really knows their own life expectancy or what will bring the end to my or anyone else's life. We can only guess based on whatever information we have at any given time.

The chemotherapy and the stem-cell transplant worked. There is no cancer in my blood. My body took a beating during the first 22 months. Other issues arise that can slow me down. They, I believe, are caused by a suppressed immunity. Things such as a foot infection, Bullous Pemphigoid on my feet and others may happen a little easier than if I had a more robust immune system. Everyone is different so others may not have the same side effects or different ones altogether. I will still be wearing a mask and taking other precautions long after most people, even when new cases of COVID decrease significantly.

Charlotte

Self-Preservation

While Mark was a patient at Grand River Hospital oncology he had many roommates in his semi-private room. Each had their own story and with such close quarters, you often learned what their story was, or at least overheard it. My favourite roommate of his was Gerald. Gerald was 82, he was mild mannered, sweet, gentlemanly, and he had the same first name as my own father. Gerald was having outpatient radiation for some form of stomach or gastrointestinal cancer but he had started throwing up blood so they called 911. He was going to be okay in the short term but he was scared. His wife came daily but never stayed very long. She often brought her sister in law with her. They conversed about many things, but rarely Gerald's health or how he was feeling. She always left by 3 in the afternoon to go home to have dinner and watch the hockey game. He would cry when she went to leave which always made her hasten her departure, telling him from the doorway to picture his happy place. Once, it made me cry too. I wanted to go over and hug him, just listen to him talk about what was scaring him and how he was feeling and let him know he wasn't alone. Mark was still here, very much alive and I could talk with him, kiss him, hold his hand, laugh with him and tell him I loved him - why wouldn't everyone else's spouse on this ward want to do the same?! I suppose my lack of understanding of his wife's reaction and behaviour came across as condemnation. Meara quickly pointed out Gerald's wife was self preserving. In fact, her reaction to the situation was perfectly normal according to Meara, psychological theory and a large proportion of the population. Apparently it was I who was the atypical one, spending 12-14 hours at the hospital every day with Mark, keeping a binder of notes from every conversation with the doctors, and supporting his care in any non medical way I could such as getting him ice water or changing his bed.

From the day of his diagnosis to the present, and his recuperation at home, we spend an inordinate amount of time in each other's company. I very rarely tire of this, and I never tire of looking into his soulful blue eyes or holding his hand. I have come to realize my spending countless hours at his bedside is my own way of self preserving. At this early point in our journey I believed he was going to make it; he would survive his diagnosis of Leukemia. I am not stupid; I heard the doctors' as they shared the odds, the percentage rates of survival and the long term prognosis. But thinking and questioning whether he could beat the odds meant there was doubt. Just like looking where your car is going when you skid on ice instead of looking where you want your car to be going often leads to being stranded in a ditch, I had to believe Mark was going to be in the percentage that made it regardless of what the number was- some people survived and I had no reason to think he wouldn't be one of them. My self preservation strategy also ensured that if things did not go as I hoped and wanted - he didn't survive- Mark would know how much I loved him, and that I had done everything I could to try and save him. So, my self preservation was based on not having to live with any guilt. The concept of having to rebuild my life without him was an insurmountable idea. As my opening sentence states, I have cried every day this past year.

Charlotte

July 30, 2021 is the one year anniversary since the transplant (1:13 p.m. exactly as I have a photo of the first vial of stem cells being transfused). It has been such an unbelievable roller coaster of a year since transplant, and the previous 6 months before that as well. I look back and reflect on how far Mark has come physically, mentally and health wise in general. I am not the same person I was on February 1, 2020, for better or for worse. There are many decisions and actions I took which I second guess now, and some I regret, but there is no script, no playbook you can follow when your spouse is diagnosed with acute leukemia. The past 18 months have felt very much like a fight - a fight to keep Mark alive and get him better at any cost - for myself so I can only imagine how Mark has felt about the numerous procedures and medications and the accompanying highs and lows of both.

I have more good days than bad at this point in time. I feel like I have a small glimpse of the possibilities that lie ahead for us - moving to a smaller house, starting some volunteer work, getting a part time job to keep me in a routine. I am elated to once again look ahead with optimism to a life with Mark with endless possibilities and no timelines.

Mark

July 30, 2021 marks the 1 year anniversary of my stem-cell transplant (18 months since diagnosis). There was a "stem-cellebration". I sometimes refer to myself as Mark 2.0. At this point there is still a lot of work to do in unpacking the events of the past 18 months and getting my body much stronger. I still don't know at this point if further back surgery will be required. Judging by the way I currently feel I think the answer is yes. I hope I'm wrong. I have regular monitoring by the team at Juravinski Cancer Centre where I can bring forward concerns and have medications adjusted. I wonder how long it will take to stop all of the medications that I have needed and which ones I will stay on indefinitely?

Also, my immune system is still compromised. I have to be extra careful so I don't contract COVID and other viruses such as influenza. My immunocompromised state should slowly improve but it could take 2-3 years from diagnosis.

I am about 22 months into my journey. As I write this sentence it is now November 20, 2021.

The journey continues...

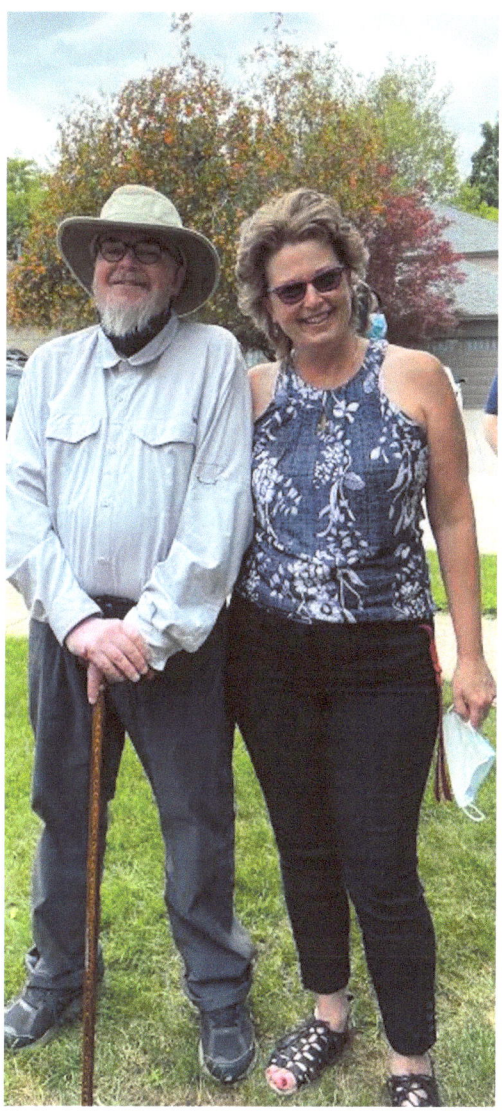

Carolyn and I on July 31, 2021 at the "Stem-Cellebration"

CREDITS

Johnny Clegg, Sipho McHunu and Jaluka, Spirit is the Journey (song), from the album Scatterings, Warner Brothers Records Inc., Distributed by WEA Music of Canada Limited, Scarborough Ontario, 1983

FURTHER READING

Siddhartha, Mukherjee, The Emperor of all Maladies, Scribner, New York, 2010

Appendix A

March 28, 2020

Dear Friends

Thank-you so much for coming today! I would love to be here. However I need to self-isolate for reasons related to my illness and because of COVID-19. I am still immunocompromised and I'm told it's imperative that I don't get a virus or infection of any kind. I am also quite weak as I continue with my treatments. I am very much looking forward to regaining energy and strength but it will take significant time.

Also, the blood drive could have been an opportunity for socializing, and I would love to see everyone. However I want everyone to be safe, given COVID-19. Please don't put yourself at risk.

For those who chose not to come today because of COVID-19, it's perfectly understandable. Please let people know that and also that blood can be given at another time, should people choose to do so. It all helps. I have been given blood and blood products through my illness so far and continue to receive it. I am astounded at how much I actually use. I am truly grateful that it is there, and it has saved my life literally. Again, thank you so much for coming today and making a difference in a person's life!

I want to thank those who organized this blood drive. Thank-you very much to Jan Laffin, and to those rallying the troops in different schools. Thank-you Jeanette Voaden and Leah Carter. I'm sure there are others out there to which I'm not even aware. You are helping give the gift of life!

Stay Safe and Be Well
Mark Maloney

www.ingramcontent.com/pod-product-compliance
Lightning Source LLC
LaVergne TN
LVHW070047070526
838200LV00033B/493